THE MENOPAUSE

REALITY

Knowing and understanding the facts about menopause

Dorothy J. Owens

TABLE OF CONTENTS

INTRODUCTION

Menopause is only predictable in its unpredictability. When you combine widespread misinformation, a lack of research, and a culture of shame surrounding women's bodies, it's no surprise that women are unsure of what to expect during the menopause transition and beyond.

Four out of every five women experience psychological or physical symptoms associated with menopause, varying in severity and disruption to their lives. Clinicians and women usually recognize the transition to menopause by the onset of irregular menstrual cycles or the onset of vasomotor symptoms, which are common at this time.

Menopause is not an illness. It is a planned change, similar to puberty. And, like puberty, we should be educated on what's to come years in advance, rather than leaving people on their own with bothersome symptoms and too much conflicting information as is currently the case. Knowing what is going on, why it is happening, and what to do about it is both empowering and reassuring.

Although more than 80% of women experience psychological or physical symptoms during menopause, both women and clinicians have misconceptions about how hormonal changes relate to menopausal symptoms and psychological conditions.

CHAPTER ONE

Menopause

Menopause occurs when you have gone 12 months without having a menstrual period. Changes in estrogen and progesterone levels, two female hormones produced in the ovaries, cause symptoms such as hot flashes and vaginal dryness. It's a natural part of aging and signals the end of your reproductive years. Menopause typically occurs between the ages of 40 and 50.

People who have their ovaries surgically removed, on the other hand, experience "sudden" surgical menopause.

Why does menopause occur?

Menopause that is not caused by surgery or another medical condition is considered natural. Menopause is defined as a year without menstrual bleeding in the absence of any surgery or medical condition that could cause bleeding to stop prematurely, such as hormonal birth control, overactive thyroid, high prolactin, radiation, or surgical removal of the ovaries.

As you get older, your reproductive cycle slows down and eventually stops. Since puberty, this cycle has been in operation. As menopause approaches, your ovaries produce less estrogen. When this happens, your menstrual cycle (period) begins to change. It may become erratic and then stop.

Physical changes can occur as your body adjusts to different hormone levels. The signs and symptoms you encounter during each stage of menopause(perimenopause,menopaus e, and postmenopause) are all part of your body's adjustment to these changes.

What is the duration of menopause?

Menopause occurs when you have gone 12 months without a menstrual cycle. The period preceding menopause can last from eight to ten years (perimenopause). The period following menopause (postmenopause) will last until the end of your life. In the United States, the average age of menopause is around 51 years old.

What hormonal changes occur during menopause?

The traditional changes associated with "menopause" occur when your ovaries no longer produce high levels of hormones. The reproductive glands known as the ovaries are responsible for storing eggs and releasing them into the fallopian tubes. Along with testosterone, they also create progesterone, estrogen, and other feminine hormones. Estrogen and progesterone work together to control menstruation.

Estrogen also influences how your body uses calcium and maintains blood cholesterol levels.

As menopause approaches, your ovaries stop releasing eggs into the fallopian tubes, and you will have your last menstrual cycle.

What causes menopause naturally?

Natural menopause is the permanent cessation of menstruation that is not caused by any medical treatment.

Natural menopause is a gradual process that is divided into three stages for women:

1. Perimenopause, also known as "menopause transition": When the ovaries gradually produce less estrogen, perimenopause can begin eight to ten years before menopause. It usually begins in your forties. Perimenopause lasts until menopause when the ovaries stop producing eggs. The drop in estrogen accelerates in the last one to two years of perimenopause. Many women may be experiencing menopausal symptoms at this point. However,

you are still having menstrual cycles and may become pregnant during this time.

2. Menopause: this is the period when you no longer have menstrual periods. At this point, your ovaries have stopped releasing eggs and have produced the majority of their estrogen. Menopause is diagnosed when you have gone 12 months without having a menstrual period.

3. Postmenopause: this is the term used to describe the period-free period of a year (the rest of your

life after going through menopause). Many women's menopausal symptoms, such as hot flashes, may subside during this stage. However, some women experience menopausal symptoms for a decade or more after menopause. Postmenopausal women are more likely to develop certain health problems as a result of a lower estrogen level.

Premature menopause

Menopause is considered "natural" and is a normal part of aging when it occurs between the ages of 45 and 55. However, some women may experience menopause at a young age as a result of surgical intervention (such as ovarian removal) or ovarian damage (such as from chemotherapy or radiation).

Early menopause is defined as menopause that occurs before the age of 45. Premature menopause occurs when a woman is 40 or younger. When there is no medical or surgical cause for premature menopause, it is referred to as primary ovarian insufficiency.

CHAPTER TWO

Menopause Symptoms

What are the signs and symptoms of menopause?

If you notice any or all of the following symptoms, you may be approaching menopause.

1. Hot flashes: Hot flashes are characterized by a sudden feeling of heat, as well as a red, flushed face and sweating. They occur

when blood vessels near the skin's surface dilate to cool off, causing you to sweat. Some women also experience a rapid heart rate or chills. Hot flashes are the most common of a group of vasomotor symptoms associated with menopause and perimenopause (VMS). Hot flashes affect more than two-thirds of North American women approaching menopause. They also affect women who enter menopause following ovaries removal surgery or chemotherapy. Night sweats are when you sweat while sleeping.

They have the potential to wake you up and make it difficult to sleep.

2. Vaginal dryness and sex discomfort: Vaginal dryness is a common symptom of menopause, and nearly one out of every three women experiences it while going through "the change." It becomes even more common after that. The vagina becomes less elastic and thinner as a result. This is referred to as vaginal atrophy. The vaginal walls are normally lubricated with a thin layer of clear fluid. The hormone estrogen

helps maintain that fluid and keeps your vaginal lining healthy, thick, and elastic. Menopause causes a drop in estrogen levels, which reduces the amount of moisture available. It might appear to be a minor annoyance. However, a lack of vaginal moisture can have a significant impact on your sex life. Fortunately, there are several treatments available to relieve vaginal dryness. Apply vaginal moisturizers (such as K–Y Liquibeads, Replens, and others) on a daily basis to maintain healthy vaginal tissues.

3. Urinary urgency: Urinary function changes in women are common during menopause. Urogenital atrophy, or deterioration of the urinary tract and vagina, is a primary cause. There are two causes for these urine changes: Menopause decreases a woman's level of the female estrogen, and a deficiency in estrogen lowers the urinary tract's capacity to control urination. Advanced age, which usually coincides with menopause, has a variety of debilitating effects on the pelvic organs and tissues. Symptoms

include an increased need to urinate, inability to control urination (incontinence), vaginal dryness and itching, and an increase in urinary tract infections. Treatment options vary and include dietary changes, strengthening exercises, vaginal topical estrogen, and surgery.

4. Insomnia: Insomnia is a common symptom of menopause, and it appears to be more common in people who have lower levels of hormones like estradiol. Menopausal estrogen decline

contributes to sleep disruption by causing menopausal symptoms ranging from hot flushes and sweats (vasomotor symptoms) to anxiety and depression; anxiety leading to difficulty falling asleep, and depression leading to non-restorative sleep and early morning waking. However, it has been proposed that menopausal sleep disturbance may be the underlying cause of anxiety and depression. Joint aches and pains, as well as bladder problems such as passing urine at night, are common side effects of estrogen decline and can disrupt sleep.

Menopausal progesterone decline may also be involved in sleep disturbance because progesterone has a sleep-inducing effect by acting on brain pathways. Melatonin, another important sleep hormone, declines with age. Melatonin secretion is influenced by estrogen and progesterone, and levels decrease during the perimenopause, often exacerbating the problem.

5. Emotional changes: The decline in estrogen levels associated with menopause can result in more than just those annoying hot

flashes. They can also make women feel like they are constantly suffering from PMS (premenstrual syndrome). Unfortunately, these emotional shifts are a normal part of the menopause process. Women going through perimenopause or menopause may experience the following emotional changes:

- Irritability
- Suffering from sadness
- Inadequate motivation
- Anxiety
- Aggressiveness
- Concentration problems
- Fatigue

☒ Mood swings

6. Dry skin and eyes: Postmenopausal women are especially susceptible to dry eyes. Sex hormones such as androgens and estrogen have an effect on tear production, but the exact relationship is unknown. Previously, researchers assumed that low estrogen levels caused dry eyes in postmenopausal women, but new research is focusing on the role of androgens. Androgens are sex hormones found in both men and women. Women naturally have

lower levels of androgens, which decrease after menopause. Androgens may play a role in maintaining the delicate balance of tear production. Dry skin is caused by a decrease in estrogen levels in the bloodstream at the onset of menopause. Estrogen stimulates the body's production of collagen and oils, which keep a woman's skin naturally moisturized for the majority of her life. When your estrogen levels start to fall, your body's ability to produce oil slows, leaving your skin dry and itchy. One of many menopause symptoms is skin drying out on the elbows and the T-zone, which is the area of your face covered by a capital T and includes the forehead, nose, and chin. Dry patches, on the other hand, can appear anywhere, including your chest and back, arms, legs, and even your genitals.

Menopause Factors

A. Reproductive hormones naturally decline: As you reach your late 30s, your ovaries begin to produce less estrogen and progesterone, the hormones that regulate menstruation, and your fertility begins to decline. Your menstrual periods may become longer or shorter, heavier or lighter, and more or less frequent in your 40s, until eventually — on average, by age 51 — your ovaries stop producing eggs and you no longer have periods.

B. Ovary removal surgery (oophorectomy): Your ovaries produce hormones that regulate your menstrual cycle, such as estrogen and progesterone. Menopause occurs immediately after ovaries are removed during surgery. Your periods will stop, and you will most likely experience hot flashes and other menopausal signs and symptoms. Because hormonal changes occur abruptly rather than gradually over time, the signs and symptoms can be severe. A hysterectomy, which removes your uterus but not your ovaries, usually does not result in immediate menopause. Even if you no longer have periods, your ovaries continue to produce eggs as well as estrogen and progesterone.

C. Radiation therapy and chemotherapy: These cancer treatments can cause menopause, resulting in symptoms such as hot flashes during or shortly after treatment. Because the cessation of menstruation (and fertility) is not always permanent after chemotherapy, birth control measures may still be required. Radiation therapy has an effect on ovarian function only when it is directed at the ovaries. Other areas of the body, such as breast tissue or the head and neck, will not be affected by radiation therapy.

D. Primary ovarian failure: Menopause affects approximately 1% of females before the age of 40. (premature menopause). Premature menopause can be caused by your ovaries' failure to produce normal levels of reproductive hormones (primary ovarian insufficiency), which can be caused by genetic factors or an autoimmune disease. However, many times no cause of premature menopause can be identified. Hormone therapy is typically recommended for these women at least until the natural age of menopause to protect the brain, heart, and bones.

CHAPTER THREE

Menopause-related complications

Certain medical conditions become more likely after menopause. Here are some examples:

1. Heart and blood vessel disease (cardiovascular): As estrogen levels decline, your risk of cardiovascular disease rises. The main cause of death for both men and women is heart disease. As a result, it's critical to get regular exercise, eat a healthy diet, and maintain a healthy weight. Consult your doctor for advice on how to protect your heart, such as how to lower high cholesterol or blood pressure.

2. Osteoporosis: This disease causes bones to become brittle and weak, increasing the risk of fractures.

You may lose bone density rapidly after menopause, increasing your risk of osteoporosis. Postmenopausal women with osteoporosis are especially prone to spine, hip, and wrist fractures.

3. Urinary incontinence: As your vaginal and urethral tissues lose elasticity, you may experience frequent, sudden, strong urges to urinate, followed by an involuntary loss of urine (urge incontinence), or loss of urine with coughing, laughing, or lifting (stress incontinence). The frequency of urinary tract

infections might increase. Kegel exercises and topical vaginal estrogen may help relieve incontinence symptoms. Hormone therapy may also be an effective treatment option for menopausal urinary tract and vaginal changes, which can lead to incontinence.

4. Sexual function: Vaginal dryness caused by decreased moisture production and elasticity loss can cause discomfort and minor bleeding during sexual intercourse. Additionally, decreased sensation may decrease

your desire for sexual activity (libido). Vaginal moisturizers and lubricants based on water may be beneficial. If a vaginal lubricant isn't enough, many women benefit from local vaginal estrogen treatment, which comes in the form of a vaginal cream, tablet, or ring.

5. Weight gain: Because metabolism slows during the menopausal transition and after menopause, many women gain weight. To maintain your current weight, you may need to eat less and exercise more.

People who are still in the menopause transition (perimenopause) may also experience the following symptoms:

- ☒ Tenderness in the breasts.
- ☒ Premenstrual syndrome(PMS).
- ☒ Periods that are irregular or skip.
- ☒ Periods that are longer or shorter than usual

Some people may also encounter:
- ☒ heart palpitations .
- ☒ Headaches.
- ☒ Discomfort in the muscles and joints.
- ☒ Alterations in Libido (sex drive).

- ☒ Concentration problems, memory lapses (often temporary).
- ☒ Gaining weight.
- ☒ Hair thinning or loss

These symptoms may indicate that the ovaries are producing less estrogen or that hormone levels are fluctuating more.

Not everybody encounters all of these signs and symptoms. Those experiencing new symptoms such as a racing heart, urinary changes, headaches, or other new medical problems, however, should ensure that there is no other cause for these symptoms.

Treatment and management

Is it possible to treat menopause?

Menopause is a normal physiological process that your body goes through. In some cases, menopause treatment is not required. When discussing menopause treatment with your health provider, focus on treating the symptoms of menopause that are interfering with your life. There are numerous treatments available for menopausal symptoms.
They include:

1. Hormone therapy(this is the most common type of menopause treatment).

2. Non-hormonal therapy

It is critical to consult with your healthcare provider while going through menopause to develop a treatment plan that works for you. Everyone is unique and has different needs.

How does menopause hormone therapy work?

During menopause, your body undergoes significant hormonal changes, resulting in a decrease in the number of hormones produced, particularly estrogen and progesterone. Progesterone and estrogen are produced by the ovaries. Hormone therapy can be used as a supplement when your ovaries no longer produce enough estrogen and progesterone. Hormone therapy raises your hormone levels and can help relieve some menopausal symptoms. It is also used as an osteoporosis preventative measure.

<u>Hormone therapy is classified into two types:</u>

1. **Estrogen therapy (ET):** is a treatment in which estrogen is

taken alone. It is typically prescribed in low doses and is available as a pill or patch. ET is also available as a cream, vaginal ring, gel, or spray. This type of treatment is used following a hysterectomy. If you still have a uterus, you can't use estrogen alone.

2. **Estrogen Progesterone/Progestin Hormone Therapy (EPT):** Because it combines estrogen and progesterone, this treatment is also known as combination therapy. Progesterone is available in its natural form as well as as a

progestin (a synthetic form of progesterone). If you still have your uterus, you will receive this type of hormone therapy.

Many menopausal symptoms, including hot flashes and night sweats can be alleviated with hormone therapy.

Is there any danger in using hormone therapy?

Hormone therapy, like all prescribed medications, has risks. Among the known health risks are:

1. Cancer of the endometrium (only increased if you still have your uterus and are not taking progestin together with the estrogen).
2. Gallstones and gallbladder complications.
3. Blood clots.
4. Deep vein thrombosis (DVT).
5. Embolism of the lungs.
6. Stroke

These risks are reduced if hormone therapy is started within 10 years of menopause. After that, your risk of cardiovascular disease increases.

Severe hot flashes and night sweats have been linked to an increased risk of cardiovascular disease.

If you have these severe symptoms, your doctor may advise you to begin hormone therapy because they are an indicator of future cardiovascular risk.

Going on hormone therapy is a personal choice.
Discuss all previous medical conditions and your family history with your healthcare provider to better understand the risks and benefits of hormone therapy for you.

What are Non-hormonal therapies?

Though hormone therapy is a highly effective treatment for menopausal symptoms, it is not appropriate for everyone. Non-hormonal treatments include dietary and lifestyle modifications.

These treatments are frequently good options for people who have other medical conditions or have recently been treated for breast cancer.

Changing your diet is one of the main non-hormonal treatments that your provider may recommend.

Exercising, Participating in support groups and Prescription medications can also be recommended by your health provider.

CHAPTER FOUR

Diet for menopause

While menopause is associated with numerous unpleasant symptoms and an increased risk of certain diseases, your diet may help reduce symptoms and ease the transition.

Certain foods may help relieve some menopausal symptoms, such as hot flashes, insomnia, and low bone density.

They are as follows:

1. Dairy Products: As estrogen levels decline during menopause,

women are more likely to fracture. Milk, yogurt, and cheese contain calcium, phosphorus, potassium, magnesium, and vitamins D and K, all of which are important for bone health. A study of nearly 750 postmenopausal women found that those who consumed more dairy and animal protein had higher bone density than those who consumed less. Dairy products may also help with sleep. According to a review study, foods high in the amino acid glycine, which can be found in milk and cheese, promote deeper sleep in menopausal women. In addition, some evidence suggests that dairy consumption may reduce the risk of premature menopause, which occurs before the age of 45. In one study, women who consumed the most vitamin D and calcium, which are found in cheese and fortified milk, had a 17% lower risk of early menopause.

2. Healthy Fats: Women going through menopause may benefit from healthy fats such as omega-3 fatty acids. A study of 483 menopausal women found that

omega-3 supplements reduced the frequency and severity of hot flashes and night sweats. However, in another review of eight studies on omega-3 and menopausal symptoms, only a few studies supported the fatty acid's beneficial effect on hot flashes. As a result, the results were inconclusive. Still, it's worth seeing if increasing your omega-3 intake helps with menopausal symptoms. Fatty fish like mackerel, salmon, and anchovies, as well as seeds like flax seeds, chia seeds, and hemp seeds, are high in omega-3 fatty acids.

3. Whole Grains: Whole grains are high in nutrients, including fiber and B vitamins like thiamine, niacin, riboflavin, and pantothenic acid. A diet high in whole grains has been linked to a lower risk of heart disease, cancer, and premature death. According to a review, people who ate three or more servings of whole grains per day had a 20–30% lower risk of developing heart disease and diabetes when compared to people who ate mostly refined carbs. A study of over 11,000 postmenopausal

women found that eating 4.7 grams of whole-grain fiber per 2,000 calories per day reduced the risk of early death by 17 percent when compared to eating only 1.3 grams of whole-grain fiber per 2,000 calories. Brown rice, whole-wheat bread, barley, quinoa, Khorasan wheat, and rye are all examples of whole-grain foods. When determining which packaged foods contain primarily whole grains, look for "whole grain" as the first ingredient on the label.

4. Fruits and vegetables are high in vitamins, minerals, fiber, and antioxidants. As a result, according to American dietary guidelines, you should fill half of your plate with fruits and vegetables. In a one-year intervention study involving over 17,000 menopausal women, those who consumed more vegetables, fruit, fiber, and soy experienced a 19% reduction in hot flashes when compared to the control group. The healthier diet and weight loss were credited with the decrease. Postmenopausal women may benefit especially

from cruciferous vegetables. In one study, eating broccoli reduced levels of an estrogen type associated with breast cancer while increasing levels of an estrogen type associated with breast cancer prevention. Women going through menopause may benefit from dark berries as well. In an eight-week study of 60 menopausal women, 25 grams of freeze-dried strawberry powder per day reduced blood pressure more than a control group. Another eight-week study in 91 middle-aged women found that those who took 200 mg of grape seed extract supplements daily had fewer hot flashes, better sleep, and lower rates of depression than those who did not.

5. Foods High in Phytoestrogens: Phytoestrogens are compounds found in foods that act as weak estrogens in the body. While there has been some debate about including these in the diet, new research suggests they may benefit health, particularly for women going through menopause. Soybeans, chickpeas, peanuts, flax seeds, barley,

grapes, berries, plums, green and black tea, and many other foods contain phytoestrogens naturally. In a meta-analysis of 21 soy studies, postmenopausal women who took soy isoflavone supplements for at least four weeks had 14% higher estradiol (estrogen) levels than those who took a placebo. The outcomes, meanwhile, did not show any statistical significance. Another review of 15 studies ranging from 3 to 12 months found that phytoestrogens such as soy, isoflavone supplements, and red clover reduced hot flashes when compared to control groups, with no serious side effects.

6. Quality Protein: The loss of muscle mass and bone strength associated with menopause is linked to a decrease in estrogen. As a result, women going through menopause should consume more protein. Women over the age of 50 should consume 0.45–0.55 grams of protein per pound (1–1.2 grams per kg) of body weight per day, or 20–25 grams of high-quality protein per meal. In the United States, the RDA for protein is 0.36 grams in one pound (0.8

grams per kg) of body weight for all adults over the age of 18, representing the bare minimum required for good health. Protein's recommended macronutrient distribution range is 10-35 percent of total daily calories. A recent one-year study of 131 postmenopausal women found that those who took 5 grams of collagen peptides daily had significantly higher bone mineral density than those who took a powdered placebo. . The most prevalent protein in your body is collagen. In a large study of adults over 50, eating dairy protein was associated with an 8% lower risk of hip fracture, while eating plant protein was associated with a 12% reduction. Protein-rich foods include eggs, meat, fish, legumes, and dairy products. Protein powders can also be added to smoothies or baked goods.

Therefore, including dairy products, healthy fats, whole grains, fruits and vegetables, phytoestrogen-rich foods, and quality protein sources in your diet may help alleviate some menopausal symptoms.

Foods to avoid

Avoiding certain foods may help alleviate some of the symptoms associated with menopause, such as hot flashes, weight gain, and insomnia.

These are some examples:

1. Sugars and processed carbohydrates: High blood sugar, insulin resistance, and metabolic syndrome have all been linked to

an increased incidence of hot flashes in menopausal women. Processed foods and added sugars have been shown to rapidly raise blood sugar levels. The more processed a food, the more noticeable its effect on blood sugar. As a result, limiting your intake of added sugars and processed foods like white bread, crackers, and baked goods during menopause may help reduce hot flashes. According to US guidelines, your added sugar intake should be less than 10% of your daily calorie intake, which means that if you eat a 2,000-

calorie diet, your added sugar intake should be less than 200 calories or 50 grams.

2. Caffeine and alcohol: Studies have shown that caffeine and alcohol can cause hot flashes in menopausal women. Caffeine and alcohol consumption increased the severity of hot flashes but not their frequency in one study of 196 menopausal women. Another study, on the other hand, linked caffeine consumption to a lower incidence of hot flashes. As a result, it may be worthwhile to see if eliminating caffeine affects

your hot flashes. Another factor to consider is that caffeine and alcohol are known sleep disruptors, and many menopausal women have difficulty sleeping. If this is the case for you, avoid caffeine or alcohol close to bedtime.

3. Spicy Foods: It is common for women going through menopause to avoid spicy foods. However, evidence to back this up is scant. One study of 896 menopausal women in Spain and South America looked at the relationship between lifestyle

factors and hot flashes and found that spicy food consumption was associated with an increase in hot flashes. Another study in 717 perimenopausal women in India linked hot flashes to spicy food consumption and levels of anxiety. The researchers concluded that hot flashes were more severe in women who had poor overall health. Because your reaction to spicy foods may vary, use your best judgment when incorporating them into your diet and avoid them if they appear to aggravate your symptoms.

4. Foods High in Salt: High salt consumption has been linked to lower bone density in postmenopausal women. A study of over 9,500 postmenopausal women found that consuming more than 2 grams of sodium per day was associated with a 28% increased risk of low bone mineral density. Furthermore, the decrease in estrogen after menopause raises your risk of developing high blood pressure. Reduced sodium consumption may help reduce this risk. Furthermore, in a randomized study of 95 postmenopausal

women, those who ate a moderate-sodium diet had better overall mood than those who ate a generally healthy diet with no salt restriction.

Therefore, avoiding processed carbohydrates, added sugars, alcohol, caffeine, spicy foods, and foods high in salt may help to alleviate menopausal symptoms.

CHAPTER FIVE

Menopause Symptoms Management

Certain things in your daily life may be triggers for menopausal symptoms. To help relieve your symptoms, try to identify and avoid these triggers.

This could include sleeping in a cool room at night, dressing in layers, or quitting smoking.

 MLosing weight may also help with hot flashes.

Other suggestions include;

1. Exercising: Working out can be difficult if you have hot flashes, but it can help relieve several other menopausal symptoms. Exercise can help you sleep better at night and is recommended if you suffer from insomnia. Calm, tranquil types of exercise, such as yoga, can also improve your

mood and alleviate any fears or anxiety you may be experiencing.

2. Joining support groups: For many, talking to other women who are going through menopause can be a huge relief. Joining a support group can not only provide an outlet for the many emotions racing through your mind, but it can also assist you in answering questions you may not even be aware you have.

3. Prescription medications, such as estrogen therapy (estrogen in the form of a cream, gel, or pill),

birth control pills, and antidepressants (SSRIs and SNRIs), can help manage menopausal symptoms such as mood swings and hot flashes. Prescription vaginal creams can aid in the relief of vaginal dryness. Gabapentin, a seizure medication, has been shown to alleviate hot flashes. Speak with your doctor to see if non-hormonal medications can help you manage your symptoms.

Frequently Asked Questions

~What exactly are hot flashes, and how long will they last?

One of the most common menopausal symptoms is hot flashes. It's a brief feeling of warmth. Hot flashes aren't the same for everyone, and there's no clear cause for them. Aside from the heat, hot flashes may be accompanied by a red flushed face, sweating, feeling hot after you feel chilled, etc.

Hot flashes not only feel differently for each individual, but they can also last for varying lengths of time. Some women only experience hot flashes for a short time during menopause. Others may suffer from hot flashes for the rest of their lives. Hot flashes usually get less severe as time passes. Hot flashes vary in intensity, frequency, and duration depending on the individual.

~What is the cause of a hot flash?

A hot flash can be triggered by a variety of everyday activities. Caffeine

is one of the things to watch out for.
Others include;

- ☒ Smoking and caffeine intake
- ☒ Spicy foods
- ☒ Alcohol
- ☒ Tight outfits
- ☒ Stress and worry
- ☒ Hot weather

~Can facial hair grow during menopause?

Yes, increased facial hair growth is a sign of menopause. The hormonal changes that your body experiences during menopause can cause several physical changes, including more facial hair than you may have had previously. This is because testosterone is more abundant than estrogen. Waxing or using other hair removers may be options if facial hair becomes an issue for you.

~Is having trouble concentrating and forgetting a normal part of menopause?

Unfortunately, concentration and minor memory issues are common during menopause. Though this does not happen to everyone, it is possible. Call your doctor if you are experiencing memory problems during menopause. Several activities have been shown to stimulate the brain and aid in memory rejuvenation.

Doing crossword puzzles and other mentally stimulating activities such as reading and solving math problems are examples of these activities.

Remember that depression and anxiety can both have an impact on your memory. These symptoms may be associated with menopause.

~Is depression caused by menopause?

Your body experiences a number of changes throughout menopause. Hormone levels are extreme, you may not sleep well due to hot flashes, and you may experience mood swings. Anxiety and fear may also be present at this time. All of these elements can contribute to depression.

Consult your healthcare provider if you are experiencing any of the symptoms of depression.

During your conversation, your provider will explain different types of treatment and ensure that you don't have another medical condition that is causing your depression.

Thyroid issues can sometimes be the source of depression.

~Is there anything else that can happen emotionally during menopause?

Menopause can result in several emotional changes, including fatigue and insomnia, inability to concentrate and a lack of motivation, anxiety, depression, mood swings, tension, headaches, irritability and aggression.

All of these emotional changes can occur before or after menopause. You've probably encountered some of them in your life.

It is possible to manage emotional changes during menopause, but it is difficult.

Your doctor may be able to prescribe a medication to help you (hormone therapy or an antidepressant). It may also help to know that the feelings you are experiencing have a name. When dealing with these emotional changes during menopause, support groups and counseling can be helpful.

~Can I conceive during menopause?

Once you are postmenopausal and have been without your period for a year, the possibility of pregnancy vanishes (assuming there is no other medical condition for the lack of menstrual bleeding).

You can, however, become pregnant during the menopause transition (perimenopause).

If you do not want to become pregnant, you should continue to use birth control until you have reached menopause.

Before discontinuing contraception, consult with your doctor.

Because of a decline in fertility, getting pregnant can be difficult for some people in their late 30s and 40s.

If becoming pregnant is your goal, some fertility-enhancing treatments and techniques can assist you. Make sure to discuss these options with your healthcare provider.

~What effect does menopause have on my bladder control?

Unfortunately, bladder control issues (also known as urinary incontinence) are common in menopausal women. There are several reasons for this, including:

a. Estrogen: This hormone has several functions in your body. Not only does estrogen regulate your period and promote changes in your body during pregnancy, but it also protects the lining of your bladder and urethra.

b. Pelvic floor muscles: These muscles support the organs in your pelvis, specifically your bladder and uterus. Over time, these muscles may degenerate. This can occur during pregnancy, childbirth, or as a result of weight gain. Urinary incontinence can occur when the muscles weaken (leakage).

You may experience the following bladder control issues:

a. Incontinence due to stress (leakage when you cough, sneeze or lift something heavy).
b. Urge urinary incontinence (leakage because your bladder squeezes at the wrong time).

c. Urination that hurts (discomfort each time you urinate).

d. Nocturia (feeling the need to wake up in the night to urinate).

~Do men experience menopause?

Andropause, also known as male menopause, refers to a decline in testosterone levels in men. Testosterone production in men declines at a much slower rate than estrogen production in women, at about 1% per year.

Because it is not as drastic a hormonal shift and does not have the same intensity of side effects as menopause in women, healthcare providers frequently debate whether to call this slow decline in testosterone menopause.

Because the change occurs over many years or decades, some men will not even notice it.

The male version of menopause is also known as age-related low testosterone, male hypogonadism, or androgen deficiency.

~Will a hysterectomy cause me to enter menopause?

The uterus is removed during a hysterectomy. After this procedure, you will not have a period. However, if you kept your ovaries (removal of your ovaries is known as an oophorectomy), you may not experience symptoms of menopause right away. If your ovaries are also removed, you will experience menopausal symptoms immediately.

<u>Reasons to Look Forward to</u>

<u>Menopause</u>

If you're like many women, you might be surprised to learn that menopause can bring about positive changes in your life.

Menopause is usually associated with a slew of unpleasant symptoms, including hot flashes, vaginal dryness, mood swings, thinning hair, and sleep disturbances. The list is long and depressing.

Menopause, on the other hand, can have a positive impact on your life; for example, not all physical changes caused by decreased female hormone levels are negative.

For another thing, many emotional and social changes can be energizing. Continue reading to discover what many women have already discovered: Menopause can be a welcome change in many ways.

1. Menopause marks the end of the menstrual cycle, which for many women is cause for celebration in and of itself. It means no more fiddling with tampons or pads, no more worrying about leakage, and no more cramping during menstruation. And, after the perimenopausal years, when periods frequently become irregular and bleeding may be heavy, it eliminates the guessing game of when your period will begin or end. On days when the bleeding is severe, some women are even restricted to their

homes. Menopause can be extremely liberating for them.

2. Say goodbye to PMS: Premenstrual syndrome (PMS) can cause a slew of physical and emotional symptoms in the week or two before your period, ranging from breast tenderness and headache pain to food cravings and irritability. PMS is a very common condition. According to the American College of Obstetricians and Gynecologists, at least 85% of menstruating women experience one or more symptoms each

month. PMS can worsen temporarily during perimenopause as estrogen levels rise and fall. So it's all the better if PMS goes away after menopause. Perimenopause involves a number of years of a very rough hormonal ride, so there's no doubt that menopause can be a 'Ahhhh!' kind of time, especially for women who have had mood changes around these hormonal fluxes.

3. Sex Without Pregnancy Concerns: Women in menopause can enjoy sex without worrying about

pregnancy. According to the Study of Women's Health Across the Nation, a multisite, longitudinal study of the physical and psychosocial changes women experience in midlife, including menopause, this makes a significant difference. Sex without thinking about pregnancy was frequently cited as one of the benefits of menopause by American women of various ethnic groups. Some women even find that once they reach menopause, they can enjoy sex more because they no longer have to worry about the unexpected outcome.

4. The End of Hormonal Headaches: According to the National Headache Foundation, women experience migraines three times more frequently than men. Menstrual migraines, or headaches that coincide with ovulation and menstruation, affect roughly 70% of these women. These headaches, like other migraines, cause throbbing pain on one side of the head, and are sometimes accompanied by nausea, vomiting, and light or

sound sensitivity. During a normal menstrual cycle, fluctuating levels of the hormones estrogen and progesterone can cause menstrual migraines. However, estrogen and progesterone levels fall after menopause, and the number of hormonal headaches often decreases as well. Headaches may temporarily worsen during the turbulent hormone changes associated with perimenopause, but migraine sufferers can expect relief once they have passed through the menopause transition.

5. Uterine Fibroids Shrink: Many women in their 50s develop fibroids, which are benign uterine tumors. Fibroids develop when estrogen levels in the body are high, such as during pregnancy, when estrogen and progesterone levels rise, and during perimenopause, when estrogen levels fluctuate from low to high. Doctors may recommend surgery if fibroid symptoms such as pain, heavy menstrual bleeding, and bladder pressure are severe. Fortunately, fibroids usually stop growing or shrink when women

reach menopause and their estrogen levels drop. Menopause is welcome for women who have been tracking fibroid growth in order to avoid surgery, or for those who have heavy periods due to fibroids. Menopause is a relief for women who have fibroids on their bladder!

6. A Chance to Reflect: This is described as the surge of energy, both physical and psychological, that some women experience following menopause. As a result, menopause is a natural time for women to reflect on their lives.

Many people decide to reconsider their relationships, professions, ways of caring for their own health, and how they want to spend their energy. It's critical to use this wake-up call to say, 'Let's put our best foot forward as we move forward.' You can ask yourself if you're heading in the right direction, both professionally and personally, and if the way you spend your time is meaningful to you.

7. Greater Self-Assurance: It's common for postmenopausal women to report feeling

empowered, which is due in part to the biological changes that occur during menopause and in part to the stage of life at which menopause occurs. Women are frequently relieved to no longer have monthly periods, which carry the risk of pregnancy, mood swings, and other PMS symptoms. Simultaneously, your children are growing older, freeing you to pursue your professional and personal goals. Women are more likely to go after what they want after 50 years of life experience, including the ups and downs of relationships, child-rearing, and careers.

8. A Time to Take Chances: People say that after menopause, you only have a third of your life left, but I tell women, "You only have half of your life left." Stop being so reserved because the party is about to begin.' This is a message that menopausal women are primed to hear, because midlife is when women are more likely to take risks. Some people change careers, or turn a hobby into a business. Others experiment with online dating or other daring

activities such as mountain climbing or figure skating. If you've been putting something off, there's no better time than the present to experience what life has to offer.

9. Focus on Self-Care: With children grown or on their way to independence and a well-established career, women in menopause have more time to care for themselves. There has never been a better time for a health makeover. Many menopausal women are open to making changes that will help

them maintain or improve their health. These changes can begin with routine health checkups and screenings, such as mammograms and Pap tests. You can also put your best foot forward by eating a healthy diet high in fruits and vegetables and getting regular physical activity, which can include anything from walking and biking to gardening and housework. Finally, it is critical to de-stress by using techniques such as meditation, relaxation techniques, or tai chi.

10.   Bonding With Other Menopausal Women: When hot flashes have you peeling layers of clothing off or you can't remember what you came to the supermarket for, you're likely to feel kinship with any other woman who is sweaty or forgetful like you. Talking and joking with other women about your menopausal symptoms can be very helpful in reassuring you that you're not alone. In addition to sharing coping mechanisms, sympathies, and empathy, women who share their tales get the confidence to face the world

because they know that they are not alone and that undesirable symptoms will pass.